How to fight insomnia

A final solution.

Hello and welcome to my book on how to fight insomnia and start sleeping well; to start let's begin with the basics,

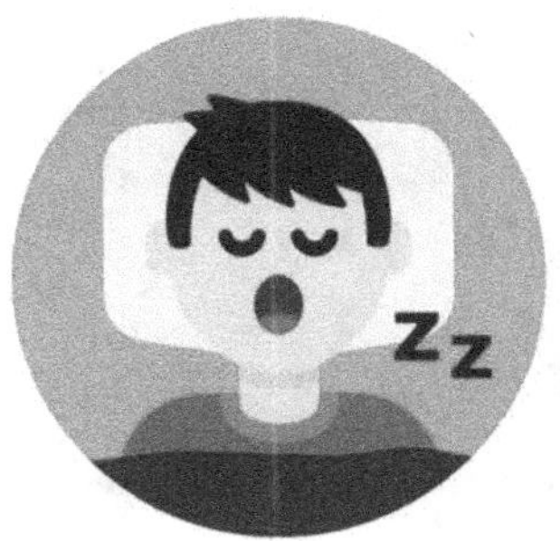

What is insomnia?:

Insomnia, also known as sleeplessness, is a sleep disorder in which people have trouble
sleeping. They may have difficulty falling asleep, or staying asleep as long as desired.
Insomnia is typically followed by daytime sleepiness, low energy, irritability, and a
depressed mood.

What is the main cause of insomnia?:

*Common causes of chronic insomnia include: Stress.
Concerns about work, school, health,
finances or family can keep your mind active at
night, making it difficult to sleep.
Stressful life events or trauma such as the death or
illness of a loved one, divorce,
or a job loss also may lead to insomnia.*

Insomnia and the Dangers of Not Enough Sleep:

You risk injury at home, work and on the road. Regular poor sleep puts you at risk for
some serious medical conditions, including obesity, heart disease and diabetes.
The continued lack of sleep can cause high blood pressure (hypertension). Depression
and other mood disorders are linked to lack of sleep.

If you find yourself tossing and turning most nights, unable to fall asleep, you're in good company.

Insomnia, which is twice as common in women as in men, affects 7% to 12% of adults. It's the most common sleep disorder.

Yet often goes undiagnosed and untreated, according to a new report. The consequences can be much more serious than daytime sleepiness.

Research has linked insomnia to high blood pressure, congestive heart failure, diabetes, and other ailments.

Public awareness of insomnia has grown in recent years, Although there's no standard definition for insomnia, suggested criteria include taking more than 30 minutes to fall asleep, waking up too early, or sleeping less than 6.5 hours a night, if you meet any of those criteria and feel like you can't focus during the day because you're so tired, you might have insomnia, they say. But if you feel fine after sleeping less than 6.5 hours at night, you might just be a short sleeper.

*I myself suffered a chronic insomnia since my early days,
i was around 12 years old when i started noticing
everyone was sleeping but not me.*

*Every single night i was not capable of sleeping like
normal people, i didnt really care about in until i got into
college where i started sleeping during
class hours, and having bad mood and feeling tired all the
day, not having appetite at all, which in result let to weight
loss bad grades in college
super bad mood swings.*

I will give MY you 10 suggested tips to fight insomnia:

1-Wake up at the same time each day; It is tempting to sleep late on weekends, especially if you have had poor sleep during the week. However,

if you suffer from insomnia you should get up at the same time every day in order to train your body to wake at a consistent time.

2- Eliminate alcohol and stimulants like nicotine and caffeine; The effects of caffeine can last for several hours, perhaps up to 24 hours,
so the chances of it affecting sleep are significant. Caffeine may not only cause difficulty initiating sleep, but may also cause frequent awakenings.
 Alcohol may have a sedative effect for the first few hours following consumption, but it can then lead to frequent arousals and a non-restful night's sleep.
 If you are on medications that act as stimulants, such as decongestants or asthma inhalers, ask your doctor when they should best be taken to help minimize any affect on sleep.

3-Exercise regularly; Regular exercise can improve sleep quality and duration. However, exercising immediately before bedtime can have a stimulant effect on the
body and should be avoided. Try to finish exercising at least three hours before you plan to retire for the night.

4-Limit naps; While napping seems like a proper way to catch up on missed sleep, it is not always so. It is important to establish and maintain a regular
 sleep pattern and train oneself to associate sleep with cues like darkness and a consistent bedtime. Napping can affect the quality of nighttime sleep.

5-Limit activities in bed; The bed is for sleeping and having sex and that's it. If you suffer from insomnia, do not balance the checkbook, study,
 or make phone calls, for example, while in bed or even in the bedroom, and avoid watching television or listening to the radio. All these activities
 can increase alertness and make it difficult to fall asleep.

6-Do not eat or drink right before going to bed; Eating a late dinner or snacking before going to bed can activate the digestive system and keep you up.

7-Make your sleeping environment comfortable;
Temperature, lighting, and noise should be
controlled to make the bedroom conducive to
falling (and staying) asleep.
Your bed should feel comfortable and if you have
a pet that sleeps in the room with you, consider
having the pet sleep somewhere else if it tends to
make noise in the night.

8- Reduce stress. There are a number of relaxation
therapies and stress reduction methods you may want
to try to relax the mind and the body before going to
bed.
Examples include progressive muscle relaxation
(perhaps with audio tapes), deep breathing techniques,
imagery, meditation, and biofeedback.

9- Get all your worrying over with before you go to bed. If you find you lay in bed thinking about tomorrow, consider setting aside a period of time perhaps after dinner
 to review the day and to make plans for the next day. The goal is to avoid doing these things while trying to fall asleep. It is also useful to make a list of, say, work-related tasks
 for the next day before leaving work. That, at least, eliminates one set of concerns.

10- STOP USING THE PHONE, a simple step put the phone away at 20h:00 /   8:00 p.m

Three more ideas for insomniacs:

There are three other things I would add from my own experience of insomnia. Meditation helps in two ways. Firstly, a half-hour session in the middle of
the evening can really slow the heart rate and make you feel sedate. I'm told that after a few months, meditation can actually induce neurological change.
Secondly, when you're lying there wondering how to slip off, some breathing exercises, in which you fill your mind with observation of the breath coming
and going, can usefully divert the restless mind. Stop thinking. It's really hard to do. But if you can just stop the mind from broadcasting its peculiar mix of propaganda, impression, recollection, projection, apprehension and sedition, you invite in a nothingness that is a close cousin of sleep.

Acceptance. The hardest, but most valuable
lesson of all. Essentially it boils down to this: bad
things happen to us, but they are nothing
compared to
 the bad things we do to ourselves. We make
things worse by our constant value judgments ("I
should be asleep"), our ceaseless comparison of
ourselves
 to others ("my wife and kids are asleep, why
aren't I?"), and our unrelenting standards for
ourselves ("If I don't get eight hours' sleep, I'll be
a wreck tomorrow").
 Acceptance is about seeing those statements for
what they are: unhelpful interventions in what is
already a tricky situation.

We are who we are, and no amount of fretting –
particularly at 1.30 in the morning – will help. What if
instead we were
able to say: "I'm not sleeping too well at the moment,
but it won't hurt me. My body will sleep when it needs
to again. I can always
 catch up." I can safely say that every time I lie awake
agonizing that if I don't sleep it means I'm not as well
as I think I am, I will not sleep.
 Whereas if every night I lie and think: I am what I am
and there is little I can do about it, sleep comes more
easily.

THANK YOU